The 5 Must-Know Tips for Nurses:

To Feel Prepared and Confident When Working with Domestic Violence Victims

Marissa F. Cohen

The 5 Must-Know Tips for Nurses:
To Feel Prepared and Confident When Working with Domestic Violence Victims
Publisher: Marissa F. Cohen
www.MarissaFayeCohen.com/Publishing-Services
Publication Date: May 27, 2022
©2022 by Marissa F. Cohen - All Rights Reserved
Printed in USA
ISBN 10: 9798832380506

ALL RIGHTS RESERVED.

No part of this book or its associated ancillary materials may be reproduced or transmitted in any form by any means including, but not limited to electronic, mechanical, or information storage and retrieval systems – except in the case of brief quotations embodied in critical reviews and articles – photocopying, or recording without the written permission of the author.

DISCLAIMER AND/OR LEGAL NOTICES

While all attempts have been made to verify information provided in this book and its ancillary materials, neither the author or publisher assumes any responsibility for errors, inaccuracies or omissions and is not responsible for any financial loss by customer in any manner. Any slights of people or organizations are unintentional. If advice concerning legal, financial, accounting or related matters is needed, the services of a qualified professional should be sought. This book and its associated ancillary materials, including verbal and written training, is not intended for use as a source of legal, financial or accounting advice. You should be aware of the various laws governing business transactions or other business practices in your particular geographical location.

EARNINGS & INCOME DISCLAIMER

With respect to the reliability, accuracy, timeliness, usefulness, adequacy, completeness, and\or suitability of information provided in this book, Marissa F. Cohen, Marissa F. Cohen, LLC, its partners and associates, affiliates, consultants, and\or presenters make no work warranties, guarantees, representations, or claims of any kind.

Readers results will vary depending on a number of factors. Any and all claims or representations as to income earnings are not to be considered as average earnings. Testimonials are not representative. This book and all products and services are for educational and informational purposes only. Use caution and see the advice of qualified professionals. Check with your accountant, attorney or professional advisor before acting on this for any information. You agree that Marissa F. Cohen, and/or Marissa F. Cohen, LLC, is not responsible for the success or failure of your personal, business, health or financial decisions relating to any information presented by Marissa F. Cohen, Marissa F. Cohen, LLC, or company products/services. Earnings potential is entirely dependent on the efforts, skills and application of the individual person.

Any examples, stories, references, or case studies are for illustrative purposes only and should not be interpreted as testimonies and\or examples of what reader and/or consumers can generally expect from the information. No representation in any part of this information, materials, and or seminar trainings are guarantees or promises for actual performance. Any statements, strategies, concepts, techniques, exercises and ideas in the information, materials and\or seminar training offered or simply opinion or experience, and that should not be misinterpreted as promises, typical results or guarantees (expressed or implied). The author and publisher (Marissa F. Cohen, Marissa Cohen LLC, or any of Marissa F. Cohen's representatives) shall in no way, under any circumstances, be held liable to any party (or third-party) for any direct, indirect, punitive, special, incidental or other consequential damages arising directly or indirectly from any use of books, materials and or seminar trainings, which is provided "as is," and without warranties.

This book is based on the real-life personal experience and opinions of the author. Please note that the names and exact places have been changed to protect the identity of those involved. The author will not be held liable or responsible to any person or entity concerning alleged damages caused directly or indirectly by the information within this book.

PRINTED IN THE UNITED STATES OF AMERICA

www.MarissaFayeCohen.com

What Nurses Are Saying About Marissa F. Cohen & Her Trainings

"Marissa was a wonderful, poised speaker. She stimulated a lot of conversation and she moved me with her story. And the discussion about resources was so important."

— Nursing Licensure Student

"Marissa, you are a warrior and I applaud that you have had the courage to work through your hurt to help others. You are so real and I learned so much from you being authentic and transparent."

— Nursing Licensure Student

"I thought Marissa was very down to earth and easy to relate to."

— Nursing Licensure Student

"There was quite a bit of content covered. This was a great presentation."

— Nursing Licensure Student

"This was a very beneficial class and I would apply what I learnt in this class in practice."

— Nursing Licensure Student

www.MarissaFayeCohen.com

"I just want to thank Marissa for her wisdom and bravery on telling her story and things that can help me as a practitioner!"

— Nursing Licensure Student

"Thanks Marissa for coming to teach us so much. For your strength and the resources you gave us to help empower people whom we might meet in practice."

— Nursing Licensure Student

"Marissa stimulated a lot of conversation and she moved me with her story. This discussion and the resources are so important!"

— Nursing Licensure Student

"Having these insights into the multiple implications of abuse is a tool that anyone who is a mandated reporter can use to help our community!"

— Nursing Licensure Student

"I believe that Marissa was very honest and straight forward about her experiences and story, which was very helpful for me to understanding the seriousness of domestic violence, and what things can transpire from these situations."

— Nursing Licensure Student

www.MarissaFayeCohen.com

October 29, 2019

I am pleased to write this letter of recommendation on behalf of Ms. Marissa Cohen, author of *Breaking through the Silence* and *Breaking through the Silence: #Me(n) Too*. I met Ms. Cohen in the spring of 2018 and shortly thereafter she began visiting my class to discuss domestic violence and sexual assault. I teach family theory in an online family nurse practitioner program.

Following Ms. Cohen's first presentation in my class I received excellent feedback from the students. Ms. Cohen discusses a tough topic openly and honestly and provides practical steps the students can take to assist their patients. When I shared my experience with the other faculty we decided to hold Ms. Cohen's presentation at a time when all students, across all sections of the course, could attend. We have consistently had good attendance, and the presentation is recorded so that students who cannot make it to the live presentation can watch.

Some students have been victims themselves and have expressed how appreciative they are for Ms. Cohen's work and her openness in discussing this topic. Other students have never been in a situation where they would be caring for a patient who has suffered from domestic violence and/or sexual assault. These students report feeling unsure of what to say or how to broach the topic. However, after Ms. Cohen's presentation the students report having an idea of what they should (or should not) say or do. They also have resources to assist their patients.

Ms. Cohen is working hard to make a difference for victims of domestic violence and sexual assault. Her experiences and expertise at speaking will make a difference not just for students, but for the lives these students will touch. If you have any questions about my experience with Ms. Cohen's presentations, you may contact me at erkfitz@simmons.edu.

Sincerely,
Dr. Jenny D. Erkfitz, RN
Section Lead Instructor, Simmons University

www.MarissaFayeCohen.com

Inspire Other Nurses to Become the Best Advocate for Victims

Share This Book!

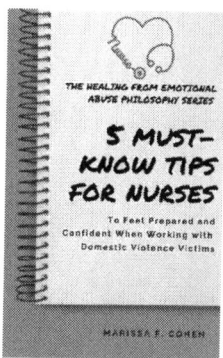

Retail: $11.97

Special Quantity Discounts

5-20 Books	$10.50
21-99 Books	$9.25
100-499 Books	$7.95
500-999 Books	$5.50
1,000+ Books	$4.50

To Place an Order Contact:

(224) 800-1244
booking@MarissaFayeCohen.com
www.MarissaFayeCohen.com

www.MarissaFayeCohen.com

Inspire Others to Overcome Their Trauma

Share This Book!

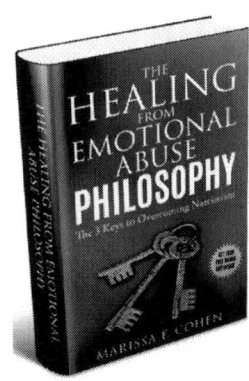

Retail: $16.97

Special Quantity Discounts

5-20 Books	$14.96
21-99 Books	$12.95
100-499 Books	$10.95
500-999 Books	$7.50
1,000+ Books	$6.25

To Place an Order Contact:

(224) 800-1244
booking@MarissaFayeCohen.com
www.MarissaFayeCohen.com

www.MarissaFayeCohen.com

Inspire Others to Break Their Silence

Share This Book!

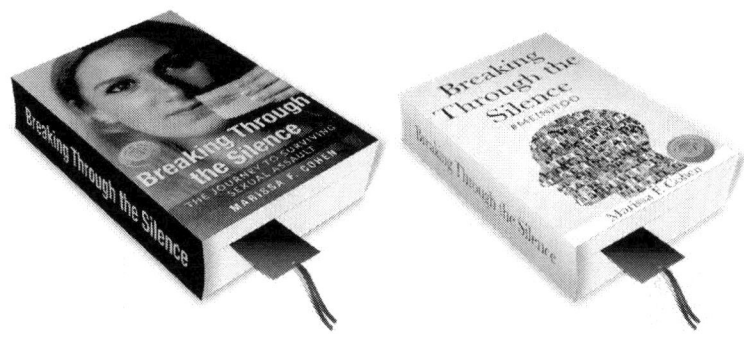

Retail: $14.97

Special Quantity Discounts

5-20 Books	$13.25
21-99 Books	$11.50
100-499 Books	$9.75
500-999 Books	$6.75
1,000+ Books	$5.40

To Place an Order Contact:

(224) 800-1244
booking@MarissaFayeCohen.com
www.MarissaFayeCohen.com

www.MarissaFayeCohen.com

Inspire Others to Live A Positive, Mindful Life

Share This Book!

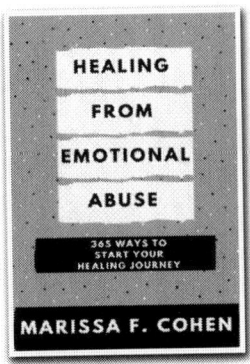

Retail: $11.97

Special Quantity Discounts

5-20 Books	$10.50
21-99 Books	$9.25
100-499 Books	$7.95
500-999 Books	$5.50
1,000+ Books	$4.50

To Place an Order Contact:

(224) 800-1244
booking@MarissaFayeCohen.com
www.MarissaFayeCohen.com

www.MarissaFayeCohen.com

Inspire Other Nurses to Become the Best Advocate for Victims

Share This Book!

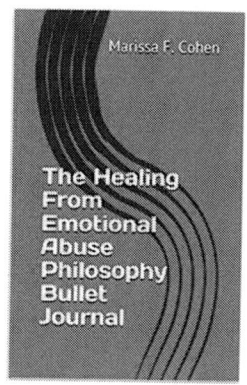

Retail: $9.97

Special Quantity Discounts

5-20 Books	$8.75
21-99 Books	$7.75
100-499 Books	$6.50
500-999 Books	$4.50
1,000+ Books	$3.75

To Place an Order Contact:

(224) 800-1244
booking@MarissaFayeCohen.com
www.MarissaFayeCohen.com

Dedication

This book is dedicated to the amazing nurses and medical staff around the world who work tirelessly to keep the rest of us healthy and safe. You are strong, brave, and dedicated, and for that I am so grateful. We can't expect you to know how to handle every case without some guidance. So this should serve as a guide to help you navigate a very complex situation. Thank you for your dedication to your patients and survivors!

www.MarissaFayeCohen.com

The Ideal Professional Speaker for Your Next Event!

The 5 Must-Know Tips for Nurses: To Feel Prepared and Confident When Working With Domestic Violence Victims

In this Q&A style event, we discuss the 5 most common concerns nurses have while working with survivors of DV and their solutions. Then, we dive into the questions and experiences they've had with patients (with respect to HIPPA) and talk about best practices to handling them. Finally, as a group, we collaborate on building toolkits for each nursing student to use, filled with resources, phone numbers and organizations to recommend to survivor patients. The goal is to feel fully comfortable and prepared to face the challenge of working with someone enduring domestic violence.

Learning Objectives: Best Practices, Keeping Yourself and Your Patient Safe, Arming with Knowledge for Better Results, Knowing Resources and Building Resource Toolkit

www.MarissaFayeCohen.com

To Contact or Book Marissa to Speak:

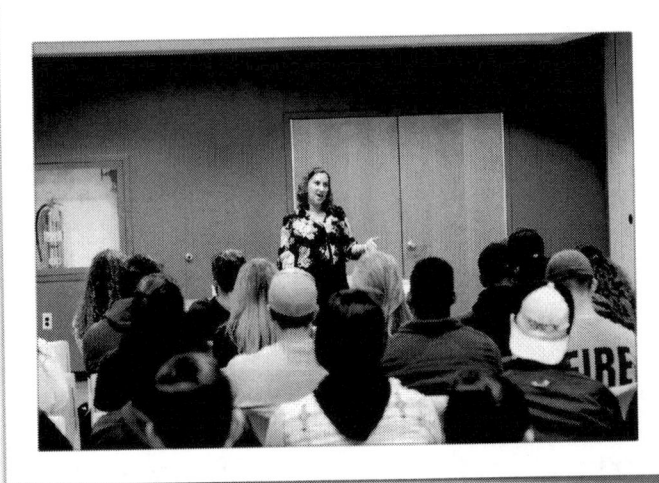

Marissa F. Cohen
1840 Industrial Dr. Suite 170
Libertyville, IL 60048

(224) 800-1244
booking@MarissaFayeCohen.com
www.MarissaFayeCohen.com

Dear Nurse,

First and foremost, thank you for what you're doing, not only for survivors, but for everyone. Nurses carry a lot on their shoulders, and I personally feel that they don't get as much credit and acknowledgement as they deserve. Especially in the wake of a global pandemic where you sacrificed yourself and your family for the sake of humanity. Thank you very much for everything that you have done, continue to do and will do in the future. You are changing the world.

The questions I've compiled for this book came from years of speaking for students in nursing schools, ranging from CNA's to DPN's.

I have learned so much hosting these programs from the incredible people who make this their living. I am so grateful to have the opportunity to partner with them, and you, and help make your job just a little bit easier.

I am so consistently inspired by the dedicated people who choose nursing as their career. The world would not be the same without you, and I am so grateful that there are people like you who help us stay healthy and live our lives.

I've learned through my work with survivors, my own struggle, and the wisdom of nurses and healers around the world the best practices to working with survivors from a nurse's perspective. These tips come from personal experience and the wisdom of people around me. Together, we've built a system that is both survivor-focused and efficient for nurses. It keeps everyone safe and comfortable.

I hope the tips in the book give you some relief, as working with domestic violence survivors is complex and intimidating. Nobody prepares you for this, and everyone will come in contact with a survivor at some point in their career. The key is knowing how to handle it before they get there.

For more information, feel free to visit my website at:

www.MarissaFayeCohen.com

Thank you for taking the time to learn these must-know tips, and embracing the best practices for care with a survivor of domestic violence!

Sincerely,

Marissa F. Cohen

Marissa F. Cohen

TABLE OF CONTENTS

ACKNOWLEDGEMENT 1

FOREWORD 2

QUESTION #1 3
CYCLE OF ABUSE 17

QUESTION #2 21
COMMUNICATION 23
ADVOCACY 26
RESPECT 28
SETTING BOUNDARIES 30
EMPATHY 32
NOURISHMENT 33

QUESTION #3 35

QUESTION #4 41

QUESTION #5 45

BONUS QUESTION #6 51
WILL YOU BECOME ONE OF MY FRIDAY NIGHT
REGULARS? 52

SUMMARY 63
RESOURCES 65
TOOL KIT 66
ABOUT THE AUTHOR 74

Acknowledgements

I want to acknowledge the incredible people in my life who have been by my side and supported my journey since October 22, 2009 and January 15, 2010. My TEAM. You have been my rock, and a big part of my healing journey. I wouldn't be where I am today if I didn't have my amazing friends, family and heart family to hold my hand along the way. I love you all.

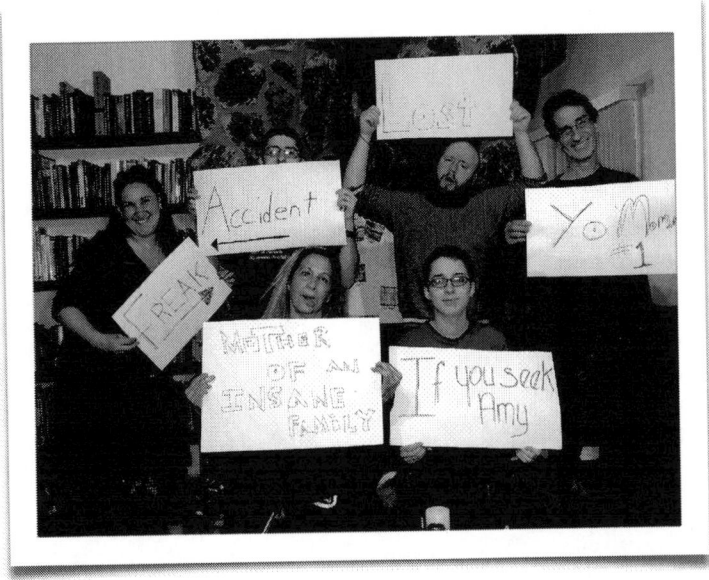

Mom, Dad, Alec, Cassidy, Monica and Larry - My Home Team. I couldn't do this without you all!

www.MarissaFayeCohen.com

Foreword

When I first met Marissa, she had just published her first book. The incredible stories of the survivors spoke to me as a nurse. Often nurses only see the bad parts and the frustrating parts – the times when victims are hurt and in need of our help, and when they go back to a potentially dangerous situation it is disheartening to us. Reading these stories reminded me that there are good endings, too.

I knew, as professor of nursing, my students needed this same reminder. Thus began a long relationship of Marissa visiting my class and speaking to my students. As I read Marissa's latest publication I was reminded of conversations with students in the past, the questions they asked her and the wisdom she shared.

Sometimes we desperately want to help but may not know where to start or how to help in an awkward situation. The questions asked in this book are familiar to many of us, but Marissa provides us with an honest answer and the background and knowledge we need to make a difference for our patients. If it helps just one person, then taking the time to learn was well worth it.

-Dr. Jenny Erkitz, RN
-Director of Nursing, Simmons University
-Section Lead Instructor , Simmons University

Question 1:

Why do people stay with their abusers? Why do people keep going back?

Abusive relationships are not as black and white as we make them seem. People who have never experienced domestic violence typically envision abuse as getting hit, punched or beaten all the time, from the beginning. In reality, that's not what abuse looks like. If it was, nobody would stay. There is a lot of gray area when it comes to abusive or toxic relationships, because it is not a logical issue, it's an emotional issue.

Abuse is a pattern of escalating manipulative and violent acts towards a person. The keyword is *escalating*. It doesn't start off one day that the abuser gets mad and slaps the survivor in the face. It starts small, with verbal or psychological aggressions, that undermine the survivor and makes them feel stupid, inferior or worthless. Abusers will continue to push boundaries and disrespect their survivors until they are forced to stop. So, after days, weeks, months, even years of being demeaned, gaslit, manipulated, and conditioned to believe that they don't deserve better, they truly believe it. Then, we may start to see sexual and physical abuse. But the misconception that abuse begins at the first physical altercation is a myth.

One of the main reasons why people stay is because these relationships generally start with a foundation of love. Abusers are known for starting out love-bombing, charming and thoughtfulness, to create the illusion that they are the perfect partner. The survivor usually believes their abuser is kind and thoughtful. That's who they fell in love with, so that's who they are deep down. When the abuser starts to show their true nature, the survivor usually just wants their "perfect partner", back. Abusers will often use manipulation tactics (which we'll get into more later) to convince the survivor that the change in behavior is their fault. The survivor did something wrong to make the abuser act this way. And survivors will often believe these

www.MarissaFayeCohen.com

manipulations because they "know" their perfect partner is in there somewhere, and will parrot the excuses the abuser gave as to why the person they fell in love with is acting the way they are. Survivors will often rationalize, justify and excuse narcissistic and abusive behavior because they, "know the real them."

- **They're just really stressed at work right now.**

- **They get like that when they drink too much, but they're not usually like this.**

- **It's the pressure they're under. It'll go away soon.**

… and so on.

Rationalizing bad behavior is very common in abusive relationships. Nobody wants to believe a person they love and respect is mistreating them. Sometimes it is from "love-blinders," and other times, it's a matter of pride.

You'll often see these relationships have created rifts or total destruction of familial and platonic relationships in the survivor's life. The survivor may have defended their abusive partner to their family and friends to the point where family and friends cut them out. Sometimes, the family and friends just get tired of trying to give advice, and help the survivor see what's happening, but the survivor decided to stay, and the family has had enough. When you aren't directly involved in the relationship, it's easier to see through the façade.

In other situations, the abuser has isolated the survivor from their family and friends by trying to prove that the family isn't supportive and will blame them for trying to break the couple up. The abuser might play the victim and tell their survivor that their family hates the abuser. Or, the survivor might realize that the behavior of their partner is toxic, but might be too ashamed to admit it. That's not uncommon either.

Regardless of what the situation is, the survivor often feels cut off from other people, or unsupported, and in turn, does not have anywhere safe to go.

Then, there are the more logical reasons...

Finances and financial abuse play a large role in why people stay. Financial abuse can be seen in several different scenarios.

1. When the abuser doesn't allow the survivor to have a job or access to money.

2. The abuser forces the survivor to work, but doesn't allow them to have access to the money.

3. The abuser will control the funds and the bank accounts, and doesn't let the survivor have any access or control of the money.

4. The abuser gives the survivor an "allowance" of what they are able to spend. It's usually a very small sum, which doesn't give the survivor any opportunity to save up and leave.

Leaving an abusive relationship is the most dangerous time in the relationship.

When a survivor leaves or tries to leave an abusive relationship, they are taking a huge risk. According to DomesticAbuseShelter.org, *"About 4,000 women die* each year due to domestic violence. Of the total homicides, about 75% of the victims were killed as they attempted to leave the relationship." The likelihood of fatal violence and homicide as a means of retaliation are heightened because the abuser feels out of control, and they will do whatever it takes to get that control back.

> *I worked in a safe house in New Jersey from 2014-2016. We took in a survivor, Leah, and her child. Leah's boyfriend was gang-affiliated, and was extremely angry that Leah decided to leave. To try and locate her, he called every safe house hotline in New Jersey to try and find Leah.*
>
> *Over the course of 4 weeks, he went to great lengths to try and get us to admit that she was in our safe house. He called pretending to be her brother, father and best friend. He had his other girlfriend, Momo, call and try to get admitted to the safe house so she could find Leah. He had his buddies calling Leah nonstop on her cell phone, trying to get her to tell them where she was, until we gave her a new phone with a new number so they couldn't reach her anymore. He and other gang members would regularly show up to our headquarters office and old safehouse location, which were in two different towns, and demand that they admit she was there and lead them to her. And so many other abusive, bully-tactics, none of which worked. We had a system in place for people like him. He wasn't the first or the last to try this with us.*

www.MarissaFayeCohen.com

We used the old safehouse location for storage and additional offices, but luckily, had moved into a new location a few months before all of this. One day, as my boss was walking into the old safe house, she found a bouquet of flowers addressed to Leah saying, "Found you, Bitch." So, that day, we advocated for her to another safe house in a different county to get her back to safety.

I don't know what happened to them after that, but I like to believe that eventually, she got out of the state and to safety with her daughter, and her evil ex-boyfriend never found her.

Abusers and narcissists are extremely controlling, and don't like when their person gets away. Encouraging survivors to leave when they're not ready or don't have a plan is putting them in danger. It's a huge risk to run if they don't have a plan in place.

And the fear of not being able to make it on their own and having to go back poses a huge risk, and a lot of hesitation. Again, leaving is the most dangerous time, so if they decide to leave and have setbacks, the most common action they take is to go back. And when they go back, they will often face punishment from their abuser. So, if they weigh out the risk vs. reward of leaving and having to go back, it creates a lot of fear. Or even the prospect of mustering up the confidence and courage to leave will most likely result in them staying. Especially if they've already tried to leave and had to come back.

Another safe house survivor story. In the two years that I worked at this particular safe house, we had hundreds of survivors stay with us temporarily, then leave to go out on their own and start their new life. Some of them stayed away from their abusers and got their fresh start. But most of them went back.

We had one family in particular that I still think about sometimes. It was a woman and her two children. She was an immigrant, who worked full time and raised their kids. Meanwhile, her husband was an out-of-work alcoholic who was also severely abusive: physically, emotionally, verbally and sexually. He relied on her to work, cook, clean, raise the kids, and serve him, and would regularly use her immigration status as a means of control, threatening to deport her without her children.
She came to the safehouse one night while he was passed out, and stayed for a couple months. She had a secure job, transportation and worked with a caseworker to find an affordable apartment until she was ready to leave. She had everything going for her.

But somehow, she lost her footing, and felt that she had no choice but to go back to him. She did, and brought the children. He punished her with horrendous abuse in front of the kids. A few weeks later, we readmitted her into our safe house. And the cycle continued.

In my two years, this particular survivor was with us 6 times. And every time she left prepared and confident, ended up back with him for various reasons, and the punishments got worse and worse.

The final time we saw her, she ran away and was adamant about staying away this time. She came in bruised and bloodied from head to toe, no exaggeration. She had finally had enough. So, when she was ready, we got her set up, and she headed out of state to start her new life, with a new job, and a place to. But it was not an easy journey or transition for her. Luckily, she got out with the children, and as far as I know, she's safe and happy.

It takes an average of leaving 8 times before survivors stay away for good.

One of the most common and heartbreaking reasons for people to stay is that they have a pet that they cannot take with them. It's the same reason that people don't evacuate during natural disasters, and why a large percentage of people in Ukraine didn't leave right away when Russia attacked (March 2022). We love our pets. They're part of our family. And leaving them behind in a place where we know it's unsafe can be nonnegotiable.

It was found by the Massachusetts Society for the Prevention of Cruelty to Animals that animal abusers are five times as likely to also harm humans. And a 2017 study showed that 89% of women who had a pet during an abusive relationship reported that their animal was threatened, harmed or killed by their abuser. So needless to say, pets are as unsafe and vulnerable as humans in domestic abuse households.

There are programs around the country that will take common house pets, like dogs and cats in while the survivor gets to safety. This reason is more logical, and easier to work around. Knowing of organizations and nonprofits in your area, such as the ASPCA, or animal foster programs where someone will take the animal into their home for a period of time is a crucial resource to have. Knowing that their pet will also be safe can encourage the survivor to leave. But again, it has to be mapped out as a part of their safety plan.

Our culture pushed the narrative that broken homes contribute to adverse childhood experiences (ACE). The mantra, "Stay together for the kids," is inherently toxic. People don't realize how much children absorb from their environments, and how much the home environment contributes to how children perceive appropriate behavior. If a child grew up with abuse in the household, and the survivor parent stays, then abuse is being normalized to that child, and impacting how that child will perceive "normal" love in their future.

Recognizing the societal conditioning while working to reframe that mindset with the survivor is important. It's difficult to undo years of conditioning, so acknowledging that that might be a reason for staying is ideal. Also recognize the limiting beliefs survivors have been conditioned to embody as well. They have most likely been told that leaving would be against their religion. It might be giving up on their family. Or damming them and their child to a harder life. All of these sentiments are commonly used to manipulate survivors and stop them from leaving, especially in god-fearing cultures and religions. If you reframe the sentiment and pose it as a question, you have a better chance of getting through to them.

I have a client who grew up very strict Christian. She married a Christian man and they are devout, faithful people. He would often use scripture and religion as a means of control. Anytime he would mistreat or abuse her, he would justify his actions with scripture, and then threaten her by using cherry-picked lines from the Bible. In order to get through to her, I had to use those same sentiments to ask questions. "Why would God want you to live with this suffering? What do you think God is trying to teach you here? Is it strength and resilience?" In order to get through to people, we have to speak their language.
However, as an advocate, you don't want to be too pushy; It all goes back to control. The abuser has control of the home, the finances, the relationship, and will most likely threaten to take the children away from the survivor if they try to leave. These threats are real, and they're terrifying.

For the most part, the legal system has not recognized the actual affects that abuse has on survivors, and when confronted with a custody battle, they will primarily default to co-parenting, which negatively impacts both the children and the survivor. So, a lot of people will stay to avoid the legal battles, heartbreak and financial strain it has on them.

Patience is key. Again, it takes survivors an average of 8 attempts to leave the abusive relationship before they leave for good. There's a good chance that you'll see this patient more than once while they're still in the abuse. They may ask you for the same resources multiple times. The best thing for you to do is be a supportive ear for them, and offer resources that might help them at their request. Forcing ideas and resources on them when they're not ready will close you off as a means of support. And chastising them about staying or asking for advice and not following it will do the same. I recognize the frustration that'll cause, because the answer is so clear to us. But cutting yourself off as a potential resource could cause more damage. So, tread lightly and with patience. Let them lead the conversation and tell you what they need.

Immigration status is another means of control that abusers will often exploit. This can also fall under the umbrella of Human Trafficking and creates a lot of political and emotional issues for the survivors. Abusers will find "girlfriends" in other countries and offer to bring them here. But when they get here, they don't have a job, citizenship or rights, and are often treated as indentured servants to their "boyfriends." They are completely unprotected, and don't know the laws or resources to leave safely. And oftentimes, the abusers will make big threats to keep their control, because they know the person doesn't know any better.

There was a woman from an Asian country, who barely spoke English that we brought into the safehouse. Her neighbor heard loud yelling and some crashing on the other side of her walls. She waited for her male neighbor to leave, and then knocked on the door to check on her female neighbor, neither of which she had really connected with before.

When the survivor came out with bruises on her face, and her two children crying, she immediately brought them into her condo and called our hotline. I answered the call.

Basically, this man had met her while traveling in Asia, began a relationship with her and her daughter, and over the course of several months, made multiple trips to visit them. And on one of these trips, the survivor became pregnant. He offered to bring her and her daughter to the States to start a life together. They came.

When they got here, he already had a live-in girlfriend, and moved the survivor and her daughter into the apartment next door. She was made to serve him and his live-in girlfriend, sit on the floor to eat, and have sex with him when he wanted to. She had the baby, which cemented her place with him, in her eyes.

He threatened to have her and her older daughter deported if she even considered calling the police or trying to leave. He told her that he was the former police chief, and knew everybody in the county, so she didn't have anyone to turn to for help. He isolated her from neighbors, and had his live-in girlfriend watching her to make sure she didn't leave, as well. So needless to say, she was terrified. She truly believed that everyone was always watching her and reporting back to him.

None of it was true. He was not the former police chief, nor did he truly have any authority or people watching her. But those threats made her feel trapped.

She felt trapped and helpless, and didn't have anyone to help her. So, when her neighbor called the helpline for her, we were able to take her and both daughters in, provide them with everything they needed, and told her the truth about her rights.

That's unfortunately not the outcome for everyone, though. Immigration status creates a vulnerability, especially for someone who is brand new in the country and doesn't really speak the language.

The best thing you can do if a patient you're working with is an immigrant or someone who doesn't have a secure status in this country is to help correct lies and misinformation from the abuser, and offer to connect them with resources they want and need. Most of the time, the abuser will have fed them information that keeps them very scared. So, by changing that perspective and reassuring them that they have a safety net and resources available to them might make them feel more secure.

*The survivor knows the abuser and the relationship best. It's important to give them the autonomy to make the decisions that work best for their situation.
*

Cycle of Abuse

To truly understand what survivors experience, you have to understand the cycle of abuse. There are three phases in this cycle.

Phase 1: The Honeymoon Phase

During the honeymoon phase, everything is happy, peaceful, loving, and kind. In every relationship, the honeymoon phase is when everyone is on their best behavior, and they are trying to impress their partner. But it doesn't last forever. In healthy relationships, studies show that the honeymoon phase lasts between six months and two years. In an unhealthy, toxic or abusive relationship, the honeymoon period will only last until there is a long-term commitment in sight. That means, once the narcissist or abuser feels that the relationship is solid, and there is a foundation built, they will feel more comfortable to start gaslighting, manipulating and abusing.

This is where abusers will start love-bombing, and building the foundation of "the perfect partner." Love bombing is when the abuser will overwhelm the survivor with acts of love and kindness, and gifts. For example, when Kanye West and Kim Kardashian got separated, Kayne began love-bombing Kim with grand romantic gestures, trucks filled with flowers, and very public acts, to prove to her that he loves her.

Love-bombing builds the groundwork for future trouble by cementing in the survivor's head that this partner is perfect, so when they explode, they are better able to blame survivor. They will use this foundation to gaslight the survivor about how the abuse is a reaction to the survivor's behavior.

That brings us to phase 2.

Phase 2: The Tension Building Phase

The tension building phase of an abusive relationship is when the survivor feels that they are constantly walking on eggshells to avoid making their partner mad. This is when you'll see a spike in gaslighting, manipulation, and verbal and psychological abuse. The abuser will usually have a shorter temper, will threaten the survivor or their pets and kids, and become easily agitated. They also show signs of grasping for control more; Whether it's by shaming survivors for clothing they're wearing, food they're eating, isolating them from friends, family and activities, or demeaning them.

This phase is meant to condition the survivor to believe that their behavior is what led to the explosion. Regardless of what the abuser does, the situations will always be manipulated by the abuser to gaslight the survivor. Meaning, it will be turned around and the survivor will be blamed for the misbehavior and abuse of the abuser.

Phase 3: The Explosion

The explosion is the blowout screaming fight. It's when the abuser puts their fist through the wall. It's when fatal threats or actions are made. It's where someone is physically abused, strangled, thrown down stairs, slammed into a wall, locked out of the house, has all of their stuff burned, the police are called, neighbors file a complaint. It is when the survivor's safety comes into question.

The explosion phase is usually when the survivor lands in your clinic. Sometimes it's a black-eye, broken nose or other easy to justify injury. Other times, you'll see thumbprints on the back of their necks, deep cuts, severe injuries, or nearly fatal injuries. Other times, especially in situations where the abuser is law-enforcement, it will be fatal.

The explosion phase is what will most likely bring the abuser to speak out and try and leave the abuse, but acting on impulse out of fear is unsafe. It would be in both yours and their best interest to make a safety plan to leave the situation safely. Poorly thought-out escape plans seldom end successfully.

For a FREE Safety Planning Kit, visit:
https://marissafayecohen.com/free-resources/
This free downloadable kit provides survivors with all the help they need to leave their situation safely, effectively and permanently.

Recognizing the cycle of abuse while survivors are speaking to you about their experiences will help you communicate with them better. The more knowledge you have, the better advocate you can be for them.

Many times, they won't realize there's a pattern. They just know that sometimes it's good and sometimes it's bad. And a lot of the time, they're grasping for the good, so they put up with the bad. Helping them realize it's a cycle can give them the ability to recognize patterns and they'll feel more compelled to get out. You are there to plant the seeds and let them guide the conversation. We'll get more into that in the next chapter.

Question 2:

How do we as practitioners best support survivors who have just experienced trauma? Or immediately after trauma? And what about someone who has been enduring abuse for a while?

Regardless of when the last explosion occurred, whether it was right before they were brought into your clinic, a week ago, month ago or six months ago, you want to treat survivors the same. There's a very simple acronym that I use to explain this:

CAREN

Communication
Advocacy
Respect
Empathy
Nourishment

CAREN covers the five most important character traits for a good advocate, which is what you as a nurse need to be. When you understand the complexity of abuse and what happens to survivors, you'll be better prepared to talk to them, treat them and work with them. It becomes less confusing to navigate. And it all starts with communication.

Communication

When you have a survivor opening up to you about their experience, your main role is to let them direct the conversation. You communicate with body language, validation and active listening. By being an active and engaged participant in the conversation, you're allowing the survivor to control the conversation, giving them confidence to speak freely and openly, and in turn allowing them to feel comfortable.

Facial expressions are universal. Anywhere in the world that you go, a smile is a smile. A grimace is a grimace. These are recognizable on remote islands and in populated cities. So, as an advocate, we try to avoid making facial expressions to survivors, because we don't want them to feel that what they're saying to us is harmful in any way. We want to stay strong for them. A part of not wanting to tell people what they're experiencing is not wanting to burden anyone. And so, avoiding facial expressions, and instead just nodding along or affirming what they're saying is ideal.

Audible outbursts in the form of a gasp, tongue clicks, or reactionary sighs are all honest reactions, but can be a deterrent to survivors. Like I said before, one of their main concerns is not being a burden. So, when you give an audible gasp or a reaction, the survivor could feel as if their story is impacting you negatively and withdraw, or feel less comfortable continuing to open up to you.

While I was experiencing abuse from my boyfriend, I tried to tell a couple of my peers one day, while my boyfriend was in class. I began to tell them, in a very hesitant and protective way, that he was sexually abusing me. The week before, he raped me, but I didn't recognize it as rape yet. I justified by believing that's what I was supposed to do with my boyfriend, even though it made me feel dirty and empty. I tried to lightly explain that to them, and they both gave explosive, audible reactions, questioning whether it was consensual or not. They were on my side, and getting worked up in defense of me. But the overwhelming response scared me, and I retracted everything that I said. I was overwhelmed by their responses, and didn't want to explore it any further. So I kept it to myself for another six months.

Body language on the other hand makes people feel comfortable. Neurolinguistic Programming (NLP) teaches us that we adopt mannerisms from the people around us, and that makes us feel unconsciously connected. For example, think about a time you were sitting across from a friend in a coffee shop. When your friend went to pick up their drink, you unconsciously also did the same. Not because you were mimicking them, but because when we're connected, our body language mirrors the people we're connected to. That's why we pick up mannerisms from our friends and family.

Do the same with your patients. Even if it's forced, it creates a connection and comradery between yourself and your patient. It instills a feeling of trust, and will most likely result in an immediate rapport, and them being more receptive to your guidance.

Survivors have learned, knowingly or unknowingly, that they are not in control of their environment or themselves. And they are usually hesitant to trust themselves, their beliefs, thoughts or memories. This comes from many instances of gaslighting by their abuser. So, by you validating what they're saying, "I believe you," "That must have felt _____." "I'm here to help you," and so on, you're helping them learn to trust themselves again.

It might seem silly and minimalistic, but the very act of being validated after a period of time where they haven't been, is like a shock to their system. You're giving them the gift of not only being right, but also trusting that their feelings and experiences were real, valid and impactful. Their emotions are warranted, which is something abusers minimize very often. It could create an emotional reaction for them, but it will also encourage them to explore their feelings and experiences more. The more you validate, "It's normal to feel that way," the more they will learn to trust themselves.

And finally, active listening. Active listening is a huge component in creating safe and impactful communication with your survivor. Active listening is listening to their story and repeating portions back to them as validation, to show them that you're listening. This isn't just a tool to use with survivors. This is great to use when children are in crisis or tantrum-mode. It makes the person feel heard and acknowledged, something, again, survivors have not experienced in a long time. But it also allows them the opportunity to expand on their story. When they feel that you're listening and invested in them, they are more likely to share. And, again, more likely to feel connected and be receptive to resources. It all starts with communication.

Advocacy

Advocacy is about support. Being an advocate is about helping that person get what they need, at their pace. It's allowing the survivor to maintain control of their situation and its outcome without feeling pressured or forced.

As a nurse and an advocate, you have a very important job. There is a chance you're the first person this survivor has talked to about their abuse. The first interaction with someone after disclosing is critical. It determines whether or not that person will reach out or disclose again.

As I mentioned earlier, my first experience trying to tell friends of mine scared me so much that I didn't talk about it again for six months. I felt like a burden, and that I might have been overreacting, so I back-peddled. That's what we want to avoid.

So, in conjunction with communicating in a healthy and calm way, you also want to be on their team, and let them know that. Even if you've experienced this yourself and you know what worked for you, you don't want to push your journey on them. What works for one doesn't work for all in these cases, because every DV case is so different, and everyone's journey is different.

To be a good advocate, support them and their choices, at their pace. If they want recommendations, opinions or advice, give it to them, but ask first. Let them make the decisions about what they feel safe and comfortable doing, and then give them the support they need to follow through.

There are people that are specially trained advocates (look up Domestic Violence Response Team (DVRT) and Sexual Assault Response Team (SART) that partner with or volunteer with domestic violence organizations around the country. If you don't feel comfortable being the advocate for a survivor, offer to call in a confidential advocate for them. This person is 100% on the survivor's team. They are trained and knowledgeable in the process of leaving abuse, filing police reports and applying for restraining orders and no contact orders, as well as the laws and legalities of your state. They know the resources in your area and are on call 24-hours a day to come out and help survivors.

If you are familiar with the local domestic violence organization in your area, call them to activate their advocate, and the person will meet the survivor at your clinic, a police station or hospital, and take it from there.

If you are not familiar, visit **www.domesticshelters.org,** and there is a map of all the organizations nationwide. The best way for you to support and advocate for survivors is to give them the most information and support their decisions. They have to learn how to take control of their lives again, and take their confidence back. You are an amazing part of their journey, and doing incredible work to help them get safe.

Respect

Respect is showing them that you have enough faith and trust in them to make the right decision that you don't try to sway them or direct them. When somebody doesn't respect you, or disrespects your boundaries, they are intentionally showing that they don't care about you, your wants or your needs. Disrespect in an abusive relationship can wear three different masks: coercion, manipulation, and disrespecting boundaries

Coercion is blatant disrespect. Coercion is when you express your wants or needs and someone tries to convince you otherwise by continuing to ask, or gaslight and manipulate you. Let's take sex for example. When someone propositions you and your initial answer is no (or a variation of no,) if they continue to ask or persistently pester you about it and try to change your mind, that's coercion. That's also sexual assault.

Manipulation is shifting the attention of a situation onto something or someone else. Gaslighting is a great example of manipulation. Gaslighting is the abuser pushing blame onto the survivor for the abuser's actions. A very common example is cheating. The abuser will cheat on the survivor, and then blame the survivor for not showing enough affection, or essentially pushing the abuser to do it for some ridiculous, made-up reason. These kinds of situations create that feeling of inferiority and distrust of themselves, and allows the abuser to gain more control

Manipulation is used a lot in emotionally abusive relationships to gain control of the survivor. And just from that, we can see the blatant disrespect.

The most important concept to take home is respecting boundaries. Boundaries are a set of rules or guidelines that show others how you expect to be treated, and how they should expect you to treat them. There are 5 types of boundaries: physical, emotional, sexual, intellectual and spiritual. That means that you have a well-rounded ability to protect yourself and your wants and needs across all parts of your life.

Showing your patient respect in all of these areas by listening to what they have to say and respecting their wishes is the most helpful and effective way to handle DV patients. By respecting their boundaries and wishes, you are giving them a gift. For the first time in a long time, someone allowed this person to make their own decision without trying to manipulate them or use it against them. That is the most incredible thing you can do for someone who has had all of their autonomy taken away from them.

They are in control. They are driving the car. Let them make their rule book and decisions. And if need be, teach them out how to set a boundary. That lesson will help them grow tremendously.

How to Set A Boundary

1. Start small. Setting boundaries is uncomfortable at first, but it's like building a muscle. The more you do it, the more comfortable you are with it.

2. Pick something that you're willing to defend. What is something that irks you enough to stand up for it? Make sure to be consistent. Abusers and narcissists like to push boundaries, so if they get away with disrespecting your boundary once, they will absolutely do it again.

Some examples of boundaries from working with survivors:

- I don't like when people stand too close to my face. I ask that people stand at least 2 feet away from me.

- I don't like receiving more than 2 texts from one person in a row. If someone sends me more than 2, I won't answer.

- I prefer that people don't sneak up behind me or grab me from behind. It provokes a knee-jerk reaction and I usually get physical.

- I don't answer phone calls after 8pm. I need my private time to decompress at night for my own mental health. Call before 8pm, or know that I will not answer the phone.

3. Communicate if someone does push a boundary. Don't hold in your frustration and anger, because then the person can't fix it. Make sure to stand your ground, but let them know

www.MarissaFayeCohen.com

that they did something that made you uncomfortable.

4. Be your biggest ally. The people who love and respect you will respect your boundaries. And if you communicate with them when they've left you feeling uncomfortable, they will support you and fix it.

Empathy

Empathy is the ability to share and understand feelings with another person. In this case, that means meeting them where they are right now on their healing journey, and understanding and acknowledging their current wants and needs.

The big picture isn't on their radar yet. If they are visiting you in a clinic, chances are their first priority is safety and getting their basic needs met: food, water, shelter. In this scenario, they wouldn't be in the market for mental health help, like therapy or counseling. So, insisting they try that will fall on deaf ears. And, you would also not be meeting them where they are NOW.

To show empathy, ask reasonable questions from the perspective of a helper or advocate.

"What do you need right now?"

"How can I help you?"

"What can I do?"

"Are there any resources that you want me to help you find?"

Asking these kinds of questions allow the survivor to feel comfortable and in control. It's not your job to tell them what they "should" be doing. These questions allow you to assess the kind of help they need.

Nourishment

When you plant a seed in the ground, it needs two things to grow: water and sunlight. People are like plants in that way; we need connection and support to grow. That is what you're providing your patients. Connection and support.

Connection is a basic human need. We are social creatures that thrive on connection. Look at what happened during COVID lockdowns in 2020-2022. When people were disconnected from each other, the need for mental health help skyrocketed. We had an increase in suicides and an increase in depression diagnoses.

You are in a position to help a person who feels disconnected from others and themselves. You can show them compassion and connection, which will give them the strength to seek out the help they need, instead of keeping this trauma held in.

We have outlined support in the Advocacy section. But taking it a step further, Nourishing support is based on your tonality and compassion. Your best tool is using some NLP. The tone that you speak to them with should match theirs. If they're speaking soft and calmly, you should match that. If they are feeling overwhelmed and their voice pitch is higher and faster, match that. It's all about creating a safe environment for them to open up. People feel the most connected and supported when their needs are being met, and their energy is being matched.

To nourish a survivor, you want to treat them like you would your best friend or family member that is going through this. Show them compassion; listen to them and support them. You have been given an opportunity to give this person a lifeline. Like I mentioned before, you might be the first person that this survivor is telling about their abuse. That means the way you treat them, talk to them, listen to them will set up their comfortability with speaking out again in the future. The number of doors you're opening for them by nourishing them and giving them the time, support and listening ear they need makes a huge difference in the outcome. No pressure, though.

Think about it this way: when you meet someone, they leave an imprint on your life. You learn something about yourself or what you like, need, want or dislike in other people in your life. They've nourished you or harmed you in some way. Regardless, you've learned something and grown as a person.

That's what you're doing for survivors. You're impacting their life and helping them grow. The connection with you might be clinical, but you are nourishing them by providing insight and help, as well as being a listening ear that can help encourage them, and empower them.

Question 3:

If the patient is ready to accept the resources, but is feeling overwhelmed, what is the first step we should take? Especially when it comes to them having to report to police?

When a survivor is ready to leave, but is afraid to take the first step, that's usually because they're feeling overwhelmed by the process. If you're comfortable, you can help them assess their needs and prioritize. The best way for you to prepare for this, is to know your local, state and national resources. Whether it's the local DV organization that sends out advocates specifically for this situation, or having the National DV Hotline number on hand, the more you know, the better the outcome.

If you don't feel comfortable or confident in the legal process for reporting abuse and getting survivors to safety, my biggest recommendation would be to find out if the local domestic violence organization has confidential advocates that they dispatch in these situations. That way, you know you're handing them off to a safe place, where they will get the guidance and resources they need.

Again, if you're not familiar with your local DV organization, you can find it at:
www.DomesticShelters.org

If they aren't comfortable with that, or you don't have a local resource, the best thing for you to do is be prepared. In the back of this book, there's plenty of space for you to fill in local, state and national resources, so you can be prepared for any situation the survivor might need.

Knowing your local organizations and shelters are priority number one. Most of the survivors that leave have been financially abused, and will not be able to go and rent an apartment, or buy a house immediately. They will likely need to find free shelter. Many DV shelters are covered by grants for 30-60 day stays. Having that information and the number to call is important. If you don't know the organization, call the National Domestic Violence Hotline (NDVH). They will advocate for your patient to your local shelter. And if they would be in danger in their county, NDVH will advocate for them outside the county and get them to a safe place.

National Domestic Violence Hotline:
1.800.799.SAFE (7233)
TTY: 1.800.787.3224

If they are ready and able to find an apartment, it might be ideal for you to have contact information from local real estate agents. Maybe some of your other patients would be willing to help. Realtors don't primarily help find rentals, because their commission is significantly less than purchasing. However, if you tell them about the situation, or have this conversation ahead of time about the nature of the rental, they will be more willing to help. I recommend having the number for two or more real estate agents, just in case. And have at least one of them be female.

Many DV organizations offer free therapy and support groups for survivors. It would be in yours and your patients' best interest to have this information available if they identify mental health as their priority for themselves or their children. If there aren't any organizations in your area that offer this type of support, I would look for local coaches, therapists and counselors that specialize in:

Child Anxiety
Child Abuse
Domestic Violence
Sexual Assault
Depression

PTSD
Overcoming Abuse/Healing from Abuse

Bonus if they work on Sliding Scale. That means the therapist or counselor is flexible to work with the survivors' budget. Sliding scale therapy is when the therapist and patient work out an affordable cost per session, so the patient is provided what they need, and the therapist is affordable and attainable to them.

Another resource for you to have would be local free or inexpensive programming for children. Libraries and park districts or recreation centers might have some interesting programming for parents to put their children in, so they can take care of what they need to. Libraries send out seasonal brochures of all of their activities, events and programs. Having that on hand could be helpful to your patients.

And finally, a general knowledge of the law enforcement process. Survivors tell horror stories about seeking police guidance for DV situations and not feeling supported or heard. And although systems and protocols have changed in the last 20-30 years, the reputation stands firm.

Offering guidance to strengthen their case when they go in for a restraining order will prove to be very helpful. Things such as recording conversations, screenshotting text messages, FB messages, posts, etc., keeping documentation of altercations with times, dates and details, keeping any notes the abuser left, and so on, will help prove that there is a pattern of abuse in the home. This also comes in handy in cases of custody battles, which are unfortunately very common.

Often, when survivors call the police, it's during an explosion. The survivor just wants the abuser to stop whatever they're doing. The police handle domestic disputes with a protocol that survivors don't always appreciate. If there are any marks on either participant, it is a mandatory arrest in most states. More often than not, there is a mark, bruise, or scratch on the survivor, so the abuser gets arrested. This poses several problems.

1. The survivor didn't want the abuser to get arrested. They just wanted them to stop. So they may attack the police officer.

2. This protocol may put the survivor in more danger if they choose to stay. When the abuser gets home, they'll abuse the survivor as punishment for getting them arrested.

For these reasons, survivors may be hesitant to get the police involved. But a large part of their safety planning might require the help of law enforcement. So, it might be in their best interest for you to become familiar with the TRO/NCO process, so they feel comfortable when they get to it.

With all of this in mind, let them determine what they need and you can offer them a resource. I would recommend asking them what their immediate, number one priority is right now, and satisfying that while they're with you. Whether it's calling a shelter, calling the police for a restraining/no contact order, giving them a safety planning kit, getting them into therapy, etc. Whatever they need, you'll be ready for it. And after that is taken care of, they'll feel a small sense of relief, and you can identify the next two steps with them.

Question 4:

As a nurse and a mandatory reporter, when we see the same people over and over again but they don't want to report the abuse to the police, are we able to take matters into our own hands and report it for them?

The short answer is, it depends. Nurses are mandatory reporters for child abuse, elder abuse and abuse of someone with a cognitive disability. If the case doesn't fall under any of these three scenarios, you are not a mandatory reporter, and I would strongly advise you not to take action without consent from the survivor.

There are two main reasons for this.

1. You would be taking control away from the survivor.

2. You could unintentionally be doing more harm than good.

As painful and irritating as it is for you to watch someone struggle and not be able to help, the best way for you to help is to not overstep. I can completely relate to the internal struggle. You're a nurse, a healer. You are biologically programmed to want to fix everything. I get it. I'm the same way. It is the most helpless feeling.

Unfortunately, by stepping in when they haven't asked for help, you are taking the control out of their hands. If they were planning to leave, or getting things together, you calling the police may have interrupted that preparation. Or if they weren't planning to leave quite yet, you have just taken over their situation and made it seem like there was a problem to the abuser.

This leads to them possibly being put in more danger. If the abuser is arrested or made known of a report, they could punish the survivor with violence for telling other people about the abuse and getting them arrested.

Ultimately, we don't know what's happening behind closed doors. Maybe they aren't ready to leave yet, or maybe they're preparing to. But getting involved without them asking for it or wanting it can end very badly for them.

Instead of that, I would recommend doing some self-care. Vicarious trauma is very real and can be debilitating. Especially in a career where you are constantly taking care of people. You need to make sure you're taking care of yourself as well.

It's really easy for us to forget that we're human, too, and hold ourselves to expectations we wouldn't hold others to. That's something that we as healers need to unlearn. So, if you have an activity that helps you decompress, work through feelings, and allows you to relax, please use that as a means of self-care. It is so important.

If you don't have anything like that, or know what helps you, below is a list of ideas that have all been proven to work.

Walking	**Scuba Diving**
Running	**Playing Group Sports**
Working Out	**Talking to Someone**
Writing	**Kayaking**
Arts and Crafts	**Paddle Boarding**
Knitting/Crochet	**Being In Nature**
Painting	**Adopting a Pet**
Photography	**Volunteering**

Do something that helps you, so the vicarious trauma doesn't leave a lasting impact on you.

www.MarissaFayeCohen.com

Question 5:

How do you ask people to leave so you can check and make sure the patient is safe?

I have to be honest, this is always my favorite question, and it comes up at every speaking event or training. It is such an uncomfortable situation when you can see or sense that your patient is being abused, and the narcissist won't leave the room. I would say that every clinic has experienced this at least once, but it's interesting to learn the different techniques that are used to get the abuser out of the room.

There are two techniques that I teach because I believe them to be the strongest and most irrefutable by the abuser for why they should leave the room.

The first one I learned from the Director of the Nursing Department at Simmons University in Boston, Massachusetts. She tells the story about how a doctor she worked with would say this to get the abuser out of the room, and it has worked every single time she's had to use it.

> *"I need you to step outside in the waiting room for just a moment. I'll come back and get you. I just need to finish my assessment privately."*

This method, using this exact verbiage does not give the abuser any wiggle room to negotiate. You are the authority in the room, and they are required to respect your process. They will most likely complain, and leave the room begrudgingly. The only piece I would be cautious of is the tonality and volume of your voice. You have to sound confident and command the room, without being harsh or abrasive.

The other thing is, they will most likely be stationed directly outside the door. So, while you're using this time to connect to the survivor and ask about safety, make sure to keep the volume down. They will likely be eavesdropping.

The second method requires a clinic-wide protocol. In the office, create a form specifically to get abusers out of the room. Make It a two-to-three-page document with the intention to distract the abuser or keep them busy for about 10-15 minutes. Have it fill in basic information, maybe a few fill in the blank questions to "gather data" for the clinic. It shouldn't be about abuse at all. Just very basic information gathering. Again, this is a distraction tool.

Keep that document under a specific name, like A-14, so everyone in the clinic knows the nature of the document, and can help to distract the abuser while you finish your assessment.

In order to get the abuser out of the room, you can say, "We have this document that we need you to fill out. I'll walk you to reception and get you set up with it." Then, walk them to reception, get the document for them, and set them up in a seat in the waiting room. That way, you know they're distracted, and the receptionists can keep their eye on them. And have the receptionist walk them back so they can alert you, or tell them you'll come grab them in 15 minutes, instead of being surprised and having to abruptly change the subject. Basically, arrange the process from beginning to end with your clinic so everyone is on the same page.

Both of these methods will give you time to talk to the survivor and offer resources if they need them. Reassure them that they're safe with you and your clinic. And if you don't have enough time to finish chatting at this appointment, they can make a follow

www.MarissaFayeCohen.com

up appointment. Or if they're safe to, they can take some resources home with them.

If they want to take some numbers home with them, you want to be discreet. With organizations I've worked with in the past, we had to come up with hidden ways for survivors to take the resources and phone numbers home without being found, otherwise they'd be in more danger. Below are some of the sneaky ways we were able to give survivors the numbers they needed. Note, some of them are geared towards females or female-identifying people, but men and non-binary people are survivors as well.

1. *Nail Files with the National DV Hotline or local DV shelter's phone number on them. Contact these organizations before purchasing, they might have some to send you at no cost to you.*

    a. *They will likely also have other creative resources for you to have and give out.*

2. *Printing the numbers on small pieces of paper, to roll up into lipstick tubes.*

3. *Using inconspicuous codewords with the phone number for resources.*

4. *Hide them inside their shoes, either taped under the tongue or on the inside of the shoe.*

5. *Have them make a new, secret email account that they can collect resources to. But instruct them not to share it with their abuser and only access it from safe devices.*

Safety is of the utmost concern here, so being cautious and having them assess what they are safe doing and taking is important. They might not be able to take anything, but let them know that you and your clinic are ready with resources when they are ready for them.

Bonus Question #6

Tell a story about a time that a nurse or medical staff really impacted a survivor.

There are hundreds of examples from my personal experience and working with other survivors where medical staff and nurses played a very important role in the safety of the survivor. There is one in particular that I like to share because it has made a profound impact on the nurses that I've worked with and trained over the years.

This story is a chapter from my book, **<u>Breaking Through the Silence: The Journey to Surviving Sexual Assault</u>**. It is about a woman who was experiencing abuse and the words of her ER doctor are what convinced her to leave.

<u>Will You Become One Of My Friday Night Regulars?</u>

I've talked about my abuse with my daughters, but not with my son or husband. I've never told him, because I felt it would be so hurtful for him to know. I told my daughters that this is uncomfortable, but I wanted them to know what happened to me to make sure they knew how to take care of themselves. Yes, you should be able to do what you want and be safe, but in this world, you just never know who's a predator.

I was a freshman in college, and it was my first time away from home. I was naive; I was not a virgin, but I was very naive about how things worked in the world. I was much more trusting than I became in the end. I went to a party with a male friend of mine, hosted by his friend who was on the soccer team. I had too much to drink, as often happens in school your freshman year, and apparently, I passed out. My friend was hanging around the party waiting for me to be awake enough for him to try and get me home. The host of the party (my friend's friend) said, "Don't worry, just leave her here. I'll take care of her when she comes to." Of course, my friend thought nothing of it. After all, he was an athlete, a buddy, and a good boy from good school.

I came to, completely out of it, and knowing that something was going on. This guy was on top of me. I was so confused because I was drunk, and I wasn't sure about what was happening. Then I felt extreme pain, and boy, that sobered me up. He was about 6'6 or 6'7. I was not aroused in the slightest. He ulcerated my vulva. I yelled for him to stop, but he continued to do it anyway. Afterward, I was still drunk, but also in shock. There was blood on the sheets. He said, "I didn't know you were a virgin." I said, "I wasn't," to which he responded, "I better take you home."

When I came in, my roommate was still up. She looked at me and said, "You're bleeding." There was blood on my legs, between my thighs. She thought I had my period and was trying to warn me, but I just started freaking out, wailing, and crying. She couldn't get out of me what was happening, so she called my friend that I went to the party with. He came over and managed to calm me down, and get out of me what happened. When they realized what had happened, we didn't even know what to do. Who knew? There was no guidance; there was nothing -- this was the 1970's. He took me to the Health Services building, and the doctor asked me if I wanted to call the police. At this time, self-preservation had kicked in, and I said no. I just wanted to make it all stop somehow. The doctor said, "I will say this was obviously not consensual. This was not willing; you don't have tears in your vulva *from nothing."* I just said, "No, no, I want to go home. I just want to go home. I just want to go home."

Then, the harassment started. The whole thing couldn't have taken two weeks, maybe more. Everyone had whiteboards on their doors, and the next day when I came back from class, somebody had written that I was a slut on my door. Then notes started being pushed under my door. Notes that called me a dirty whore, and if I say anything they will tell everyone that I'm a dirty slut. I had no idea what to do. There was a knock on my door one time, and when I opened the door, there was my attacker. He wanted to know if we could go out and talk. I told him, "No. I never wanted to see your face again."

He was just standing there looking ashamed and uncomfortable, and then he said, "So, my coach says that he knows that you had another boyfriend and that your old boyfriend (who was also a soccer player), is willing to testify that you're a slut and you would sleep with anybody." I just looked at him and told him, "You just get out of my face. Just get the fuck away from me and stay the fuck away from me."

He tried to see me one more time after that. He called me and said that he had to talk to me. I called up two male friends of mine who were on the track team, big guys, in an absolute panic. Why didn't I call the police, campus security, call my dorm, I don't know. The guy showed up, and my two very large friends were just sitting there. They stood up and said, "If you didn't understand her, she said she never wants you to contact her again." I never heard from the guy ever again. Thankfully I got past that, and I was lucky enough to have no sexual problems as a result.

I'm thankful to have had support, not just from women, but also from male friends.

When I was 23 or 24, I had a boyfriend who was violent toward me. He was quiet and seemed unassuming. He had a lot of interesting stories from being a roadie with my favorite rock band. Things seemed fine at first, and then he started having what began as little hissy fits.

For example, once we were going to a concert and when we got to our seats, he didn't like the view from the seats. I remember saying, "Well, it doesn't matter. These seats are fine. We can see fine." All of a sudden, he got up and stormed off. Now, had I been a different woman, I would have thought, "what the fuck, asshole?" stayed, watched the concert, got a cab home, and never saw him again. Because I am how I am, I asked, "What, what's happening?" I started grabbing my coat, followed him and kept asking what happened and what was wrong. Of course, I was thinking, "What did I do?" because he made it seem like my fault.

From there, it progressed. He would be overwhelmingly lovey-dovey and romantic one moment, and then would be the smack-down. It was a lot of emotional abuse. One moment he would say, "I love you; I love you," and then "I don't want you to do that, and you're going to do it anyway, and I'm not going to speak to you." For example, one night, my friend asked me to be his date to a wedding. My boyfriend didn't want me to go, but I told him, "Look, he has been one of my best friends since high school. I'm not going to tell him no. He's my friend, you know he's my friend." He still didn't want me to go to the wedding, but I assured him I would come home *immediately after. We weren't living together, but I spent much time at his place.*

On the night of the wedding, I was wearing a short dress and sandals (keep in mind that this is in December, but it was a cute, appropriate outfit for an indoor wedding). When my friend dropped me off and I walked up to my apartment. I had this really wonky lock, and usually you could pull it, and jiggle it to open it up. This time, however, it didn't open, and there I was in my short dress with my bare legs and sandals, unable to get into my apartment. It wasn't that late, maybe midnight. My boyfriend lived blocks away — within walking distance. I walked all the way to his apartment, and I rang the doorbell, and I said, "It's me. My lock won't open again. The damn thing won't open!" He said, "Too bad." I rang again and said, "I'm in a dress, in sandals, and it's snowing out. Let me in!" but, he wouldn't let me in. I was starting to panic, and I had to beg to be let in. The next morning, it was like nothing had happened. I asked him why he wouldn't let me in, and he said he was tired.

He only hit me twice during our relationship. I know, the word "only" is not great because it shouldn't even happen once. The first time was after we had broken up. I went out with someone else, and he called me when I got home. I could tell he was very upset. He begged to speak with me and came over. He started asking questions about whether the guy had kissed me during our date, and was digging for information. In my mind, it wasn't any of his business -- he broke up with me, and I can kiss whoever I want. Then he slapped me. I looked at him and told him, "Get the fuck out, and I never want to see you again." He called, and called, and cried, and called, and begged, and cried and showed up with roses. He said, "What was I thinking?" and, "If you take me back, I'll make it up to you!" Why did I take him back? The guy who I was out with that night called me, and I told him I had gotten back together with my boyfriend.

He was a nice guy, and I didn't tell him what had happened, but he said, "You know, you're a nice girl. But I g otta tell you; you're being really stupid. And it's not because you're not going to date me. It's because you're putting up with this and you don't have to." I made excuses for him. I don't seem like that kind of person now, but being with someone like that chips away at your self-esteem. And yet, I was with him for another year. The first six months because I wanted to be, and the second 6 months because I was afraid of him. He started complaining about me spending time with my male friends, but then it became my female friends too, and then my family. He didn't want me to spend time with my parents. "Why do you have to spend so much time with your family? Why do you have to spend so much time with your parents? Aren't you a grown-up?" Of course, I would keep doing it, because I was not going to step away from my friends and family. That would lead to these punishing hissy fits. I was unhappy. I was not myself, and people saw it.

There was one wonderful woman at work, this wonderful, old, grandma- like lady with white hair who was always sweet to me, who said, "Something's not right. You're always so cheerful and happy. What's wrong?" I told her everything. I told her what was going on, not realizing how bad it was. She was not sweet this time. She looked at me very sternly, and she said, "You need to stop. You need to stop this right now. You need to stop this." I believe she even used the word abusive.

Oddly enough, the thing that finally made up my mind was when I got my first cat. I didn't want to be at my boyfriend's anymore; I wanted to be at home with my kitty cat. And I began to realize if I want to be with the animal more than I wanted to be with the man, that was saying something. He didn't want to sleep at my apartment because of the cat. When he came over to my place, and we were starting to get intimate, my kitty jumped up on the bed because he was used to sleeping in bed with me. Without even stopping, my boyfriend scooped him up and tossed him off the bed. And for the first time, I kicked him, and pushed him off the bed, and said, "Get Out! Get out! Get the fuck out!" I was screaming, "Don't you ever touch my cat! Don't you ever touch him! Get! The Fuck! Out!" And he did. And I thought, "If he could abuse me, but he mustn't touch my cat, what does that say about me?"

I thought this was it, and I was done. I should have let it be over, but the next day, I told him I needed to talk to him. So, the next day I went over to his place to end it. As soon as I spoke the words, "This is over, I'm done!" he started walking towards me...and I knew. I just knew. I ran for the door to try and get it open, but he got me at the door. He hit me so hard that he knocked me out. It sounded like a "thunk," almost like the sound that you make when you hit a watermelon. The next thing I knew, my shirt was torn, I was bleeding, and I wasn't by the door anymore - I don't know how I got to where I was. I started screaming and screaming and screaming at the top of my lungs, "Help, help, someone call the police, help!" By this time, my boyfriend had gotten himself together, because he saw that I was hurt and bleeding and hysterical, and he was trying to calm me down. He asked to let him take me to the hospital, and I let him drive me to the E.R. I just wanted everything to stop, for it to be over.

When we got there, the nurses did an intake report to see what happened. I told them I fell and hit my head. So, after I was stitched, the doctor asked me what happened because it said that I tripped and fell. The doctor said they had to give me some stitches, and they needed to stabilize my jaw because it was unhinged. I had three stitches on the side of my head. "Who hit you?" the doctor asked. I didn't say anything. He said, "This is not a falling accident. This is an impact accident. This is what you get when someone hits you. Was it your husband, your boyfriend, your father? Who is it?" I still didn't say anything. He said, "Do you know how I know this? I know this because every Friday night, they come in here, these beaten women. It's the same ones over and over again. And each time, it's a little worse. It's a black eye. Then it's a black eye and a broken nose. A broken cheek. Stitches in the head, it's a concussion, and some of them eventually die. They have police out in the waiting room. I'll have them come in, I'll file a report, you'll file a report, and they'll arrest him. So, are you going to become one of my Friday night regulars?"

With that, I was able to meet his eyes, and I said, "NO! Never again".

I left the hospital and went home, where my boyfriend was standing, crying and apologizing. I told him that he was not staying, and he was not coming in, he was leaving. At this point, I was so calm; I was just trying to keep control. I went into my apartment, shut it and locked it. I went into my room, and thought, "I'm safe now." I felt overwhelming relief because I was never going to see *him again, ever...or so I thought. He called and called, trying to apologize. He would go through phases. He would call begging and pleading. He would call in the middle of the night screaming and cursing at me. One night, he was down in the courtyard of my apartment complex, banging on the door and screaming, and the girl upstairs called the police on him. He sent roses to my office one time. I looked at the card, went into the lunchroom, threw the roses in the garbage, and went back to my desk. Two years later, I was in a new relationship with my now-husband. I told my husband about the phone calls, and how I would just hang up. One day the phone rang, and my husband decided to pick it up. He said, "Yep, hello? Nope. Nope. She doesn't want to talk to you. Go right ahead. It's a whole lot harder to beat up another man than it is to beat up a woman. Come right on." and he hung up. I hyperventilated and thought I was going to hear my doorbell ring, and he would be tracking me. But thankfully, I never heard from him again.*

What helped me at first, were my friends. Women didn't talk about assault, or domestic violence very much, but if you did share, somebody would share back if they'd experienced it. It was really helpful to hear another woman say, "Don't you put up with that shit." Especially older women. I got a fair bit of counseling, which also really helped. I never spoke to my parents about the rape, and I don't know if I told them about the abuse. I mean, obviously they saw it. They aren't stupid, and they probably knew something was going on, and you could see that I had been beaten up. I think that the hardest part was looking back and thinking, "Good Lord, what was I missing in me, that I would take that?" It isn't my fault. I know it isn't my fault.

You can't let it define you; what you did, what you didn't do, how you fought or didn't fight, is not who you are. Someone else did you wrong. How it felt, what you did at the moment, and how it felt in the moment is all so confusing for a decent person who doesn't want to hurt anyone else. It's really hard to comprehend. Someone else fucked up, and you got the sharp end of it, but it's still your body and still your life. It's still your sexuality. It doesn't belong to them. I don't know how we make it stop. I don't think we can make it all stop. Women can't do this on our own, because women want to be loved and desired and wanted. In addition to wanting to be respected, they want to be desired. That's why women with brains and guts and education and ambition will go somewhere and have their pubic hairs ripped out by their roots with a bikini wax. Why? Because somebody told women, it makes them sexier. You have to have men join you as part of the effort to stop abuse. All it takes is for good people to do something.

Summary

Thank you so much for taking the time to do and be better while working with survivors. It's critical that they get the care and compassion they need to set them up for success. You have the honorable role of being a part of their healing journey, and now, you should feel very prepared and confident when that time arises.

Just to summarize, the most important thing to remember is to keep the survivor in control. All of the decisions have to be approved through them. If you take the control away from them, you're setting them up for failure. You are a passenger in their journey. Let them drive the car.

You are doing incredible work, and I am so grateful for you, your work, and your drive to continue to grow.

You're doing more for the survivor community than you know!

Thank you!

Resources

www.MarissaFayeCohen.com

www.MarissaFayeCohen.com/Free-Resources

www.RAINN.org

www.DomesticShelters.org

www.NCEDV.org

National Domestic Violence Hotline:
1.800.799.SAFE (7233)
TTY: 1.800.787.3224

National Sexual Assault Hotline:
1-800-656-4673

Healing From Emotional Abuse Podcast
https://marissafayecohen.podbean.com/
https://www.podbean.com/media/share/pb-j8ptq-d5c65b

www.MarissaFayeCohen.com/the-books

www.MarissaFayeCohen.com/Private-Coaching

_____ _____
       (Resource)   (Phone Number)
_____
                    (Website)

_____ _____
       (Resource)   (Phone Number)
_____
                    (Website)

_____ _____
       (Resource)   (Phone Number)
_____
                    (Website)

_____ _____
       (Resource)   (Phone Number)
_____
                    (Website)

_____ _____
       (Resource)   (Phone Number)
_____
                    (Website)

_____ _____
       (Resource)   (Phone Number)
_____
                    (Website)

_____ _____
(Resource)   (Phone Number)
_____
                    (Website)

_____ _____
(Resource)   (Phone Number)
_____
                    (Website)

_____ _____
(Resource)   (Phone Number)
_____
                    (Website)

_____ _____
(Resource)   (Phone Number)
_____
                    (Website)

_____ _____
(Resource)   (Phone Number)
_____
                    (Website)

_____ _____
(Resource)   (Phone Number)
_____
                    (Website)

www.MarissaFayeCohen.com

_____ _____
        (Resource)   (Phone Number)
_____
                      (Website)

_____ _____
        (Resource)   (Phone Number)
_____
                      (Website)

_____ _____
        (Resource)   (Phone Number)
_____
                      (Website)

_____ _____
        (Resource)   (Phone Number)
_____
                      (Website)

_____ _____
        (Resource)   (Phone Number)
_____
                      (Website)

_____ _____
        (Resource)   (Phone Number)
_____
                      (Website)

www.MarissaFayeCohen.com

_____ _____
       (Resource)   (Phone Number)
_____
                           (Website)

_____ _____
       (Resource)   (Phone Number)
_____
                           (Website)

_____ _____
       (Resource)   (Phone Number)
_____
                           (Website)

_____ _____
       (Resource)   (Phone Number)
_____
                           (Website)

_____ _____
       (Resource)   (Phone Number)
_____
                           (Website)

_____ _____
       (Resource)   (Phone Number)
_____
                           (Website)

www.MarissaFayeCohen.com

Name & Type of Resource	Phone Number	Website	Notes

www.MarissaFayeCohen.com

Name & Type of Resource	Phone Number	Website	Notes

About the Author

Marissa F. Cohen is the Founder of the Healing From Emotional Abuse Philosophy™, and the Award-Winning and Best Selling author of the Breaking Through the Silence Series — <u>Breaking Through the Silence: The Journey to Surviving Sexual Assault</u> (2018 Readers Favorite International Book Award Winner, and #1 Amazon International Best Seller); and <u>Breaking Through the Silence: #Me(n)Too</u> (Amazon #1 Best Seller). As well as the best-selling author of The Ruhe Approach: Healing From Abuse (renamed the Healing From Emotional Abuse Philosophy: Living A Life of Freedom, Confidence and Peace), and The Healing From Emotional Abuse Philosophy: The 3 Keys to Overcoming Narcissism.

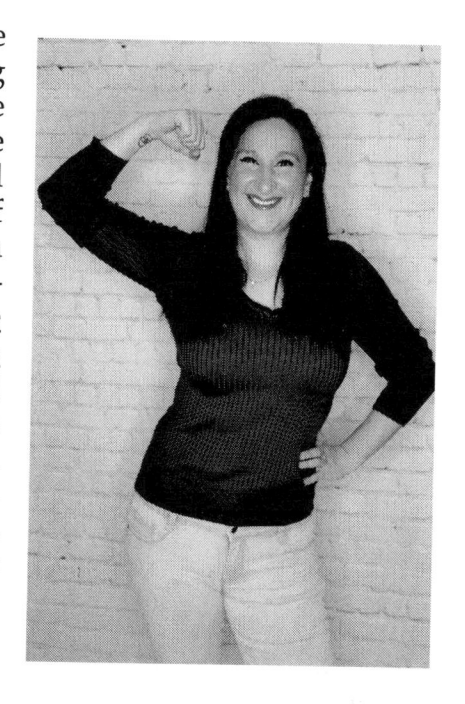

As the Founder of the Healing From Emotional Abuse Philosophy™, she has created a 3 Key Method to overcoming narcissism and narcissistic abuse. Over 2,000 people have used this Philosophy to start living

www.MarissaFayeCohen.com

a free, confident and peaceful life through her one-on-one coaching programs. It has since been endorsed by **Brian Tracy, Jack Canfield, James Malinchak, Kevin Harrington, Joe Theismann, John Formica,** and **Jill Lublin.**

As a speaker, Marissa has partnered with over 50 schools to bring DV and SA awareness to high school, college and university campuses nationally.

Marissa F. Cohen was named a Top 10 Most Inspirational Female Entrepreneur on International Women's Day 2021 by Fast Capital 360, and has shared a stage with Jack Canfield, Patty Aubery, Joe Theismann, and James Malinchak.

Marissa's Podcast, Healing From Emotional Abuse, has charted Top 5 in Albania, Top 20 in New Zealand and Italy, and Top 100 in Australia, Israel, Canada, Malaysia, Norway, Russia, and South Africa. She is also the host of a weekly radio show on KXFM Laguna Beach that reaches over 24,000 listeners.

Her mission is to empower all survivors of sexual abuse, narcissism, emotional abuse and domestic violence to release their trauma, build resilience and rebuild their lives, so they can feel complete, happy, and confident.

She currently resides in Chicago with her husband and their two dogs. She spends her downtime traveling, hiking and crafting!